Easy Guide to Low-Oxalate Intake:

Your Simple Guide to Navigating Low-Oxalate Food Intake

By

Anthony Mendoza

Copyright 2024 by Anthony Mendoza

Table of Content

Sweet Potato Hash

Cottage Cheese and Fruit Bowl

Turkey and Spinach Salad

Shrimp Stir-Fry with Snow Peas

Stuffed Bell Peppers with Ground Turkey

Banana Oatmeal Pancakes

Veggie Egg Muffins

Tuna Salad Lettuce Wraps

Quinoa Salad with Lemon Vinaigrette

Baked Chicken with Roasted Vegetables

Turkey and Quinoa Stuffed Bell Peppers

Nut butter and berry Greek yogurt bowl

Tofu and Vegetable Stir-Fry

Lentil and Kale Salad

Baked Salmon with Herb Crust

Stir-fried shrimp with Broccoli and Cashews

Chia Seed Pudding

Veggie Breakfast Burrito

Turkey and Avocado Salad

Quinoa and Black Bean Bowl

Grilled Chicken Skewers with Vegetable Medley

Cauliflower Rice Stir-Fry

Conclusion

Introduction

Your body creates oxalate, which is also referred to as oxalic acid. likewise, it occurs naturally in a wide variety of foods, such as grains, nuts, vegetables, and fruits. The urinary system naturally contains trace levels of calcium and oxalate, which usually do not pose any problems. Hard mineral deposits called kidney stones, or calcium oxalate kidney stones, may, nonetheless, sometimes result from the binding of calcium and oxalate.

This is particularly frequent in those who excrete a lot of oxalates while making little pee. Reducing the amount of oxalate excreted in urine may be helpful for those who are susceptible to kidney stones caused by calcium oxalate. One of the most popular strategies is to follow a low-oxalate diet.

Nevertheless, increasing your calcium consumption may also assist in lowering oxalate excretion because calcium binds with oxalate before it reaches the kidneys, preventing kidney stones. High oxalate diets may increase the quantity of oxalate excreted in urine, which may aid in the development of kidney stones.

CHAPTER ONE

What is Oxalate?

Both people and plants naturally contain large amounts of the chemical oxalate. It is not a necessary food for humans, and kidney stones may result from taking too much of it. By binding with excess calcium, oxalate aids in the removal of calcium from plants. This explains why so many meals rich in oxalate come from plants.

How Is It Metabolized by The Body?

Foods containing oxalate enter the digestive system and are excreted in the urine or stool. Oxalate can bond with calcium as it moves through the intestines and is eliminated in the stool. Kidney stones may develop, however, if the kidneys absorb an excessive amount of oxalate. The most prevalent kind of kidney stones in the United States are calcium oxalate kidney stones.

Your chance of getting these types of kidney stones increases with oxalate levels.

What Is a Diet Low in Oxalate?

Reducing your oxalate intake may help lessen your chance of kidney stones if you are at high risk for them. However new studies suggest that eating more foods high in calcium when you consume foods high in oxalate could be a better strategy than cutting it out of your diet entirely. Kidney stones are less likely to develop because oxalate and calcium have a higher tendency to bind together during digestion and pass through the kidneys.

Why Does Oxalate Accumulate?

Foods rich in vitamin C have the potential to raise oxalate levels in the body. Oxalate is converted by vitamin C. Levels over 1,000 mg/day have been shown to elevate oxalate levels. The use of antibiotics or a medical history of digestive disorders may also raise oxalate levels in the body. Higher quantities of oxalate may be absorbed by the body when the beneficial bacteria in the stomach are not as abundant, which aids in the removal of oxalate from the body.

What is Oxalate Reducible?

Getting enough fluids in your diet may help prevent kidney stones from developing or even assist remove them. It's best to distribute your drink consumption throughout the day. It is better to choose water over other beverages. Eat no more than 10% of animal protein since this may lead to the formation of stones. Getting enough calcium is beneficial as well. Kidney stones may occur as a result of too little calcium entering the body, which can increase the quantity of oxalate that reaches the kidneys.

Kidney stone risk may also be decreased by reducing salt consumption. Diets high in salt tend to increase the amount of calcium lost in urine.

Renal stones are more likely in individuals with higher renal tissue levels of calcium and oxalate.

How Can One Quantify Oxalate?

Food oxalate content lists might be difficult to understand. The following variables may affect the oxalate levels in food reports:

- *How the foods' oxalate levels were measured;*
- *Where they are cultivated*
- *When they are collected*

The Role of Oxalates in Health

These naturally occurring compounds are found in various plant foods, from spinach and kale to nuts and berries. They're like tiny, molecular puzzle pieces that can have a significant impact on our health, but just like any puzzle, the picture isn't always clear-cut.

Imagine strolling through a bustling farmer's market, the vibrant colors of fruits and vegetables catching your eye. Among them, you spot a bunch of leafy greens. Those leafy greens, like spinach and Swiss chard, are loaded with oxalates. These compounds play a role in the plant's defense mechanisms, warding off predators and helping the plant regulate its calcium levels.

Now, when we consume foods rich in oxalates, they journey through our digestive system, making their way to our kidneys. Here's where the plot thickens. In some individuals, especially those prone to kidney stones, oxalates can bind with calcium to form crystals, which can then accumulate and lead to the formation of kidney stones. It's like a rocky road that nobody wants to travel on.

But wait, there's more to this story. Not all oxalates are created equal. Some are more soluble than others, meaning they're more easily absorbed by our bodies and less likely to cause trouble.

The amount of oxalates in foods can vary widely, depending on factors like soil quality and plant variety.

Interestingly, oxalates aren't just troublemakers. They also have potential health benefits. Some research suggests that they may act as antioxidants, helping to protect our cells from damage caused by harmful molecules called free radicals. Additionally, they may have anti-inflammatory properties, which could be beneficial for conditions like arthritis.

So, what's the bottom line? Like many things in nutrition, it's all about balance. For most people, enjoying oxalate-rich foods as part of a varied diet is perfectly fine. But if you have a history of kidney stones or other health concerns, it might be worth chatting with a healthcare provider or a dietitian to determine the best approach for you. After all, when it comes to our health, a little knowledge can go a long way.

Understanding the Benefits and Risks

In humans, oxalates can have benefits and risks depending on various factors such as dietary intake, health conditions, and individual tolerance levels.

Let's start with the benefits:

1. **Antioxidant Properties**: Oxalates, particularly in the form of oxalic acid, exhibit antioxidant properties. Antioxidants help protect the body from oxidative stress and damage caused by free radicals, which can contribute to various diseases including cancer and heart disease.

2. **Nutrient Absorption**: Some studies suggest that oxalates may bind to minerals like calcium and prevent their absorption in the intestines. While this might sound like a risk (and it can be in

excess), it can also be beneficial in certain cases. For example, individuals with hyperoxaluria, a condition characterized by high levels of oxalates in the urine, may benefit from reducing their dietary intake of oxalate-rich foods to prevent kidney stone formation.

Now, let's discuss the risks:

1. **Kidney Stones:** The most well-known risk associated with oxalates is kidney stone formation. When oxalate levels in the urine are too high, they can combine with calcium to form crystals, which can then develop into kidney stones. Foods such as spinach, rhubarb, beets, nuts, chocolate, and tea are notorious for their oxalate content. However, it's important to note that not everyone who consumes oxalate-rich foods will develop kidney stones, as genetics, hydration status, and overall diet also play significant roles.

2. **Nutrient Absorption**: While oxalates can bind to minerals like calcium and prevent their absorption, excessive intake of oxalate-rich foods may lead to nutrient deficiencies, particularly in calcium. This is why individuals need to consume a balanced diet and not rely solely on oxalate-rich foods for their nutritional needs.

Let's take a closer look at this with an example:

Imagine Sarah, a health-conscious individual who loves her green smoothies. She adds a handful of spinach, a banana, some almonds, and a splash of almond milk to her blender every morning. While this smoothie is packed with nutrients, it's also high in oxalates. Sarah's diet is generally balanced, and she stays well-hydrated throughout the day, so she doesn't have any issues with kidney stones. However, if Sarah were to consume this smoothie multiple times a day, every day, she might start to experience problems with calcium absorption and potentially even kidney stone formation over time.

While oxalates offer antioxidant benefits and can be a part of a healthy diet, it's important to consume them in moderation, especially if you're prone to kidney stones or have other underlying health conditions. Balance is crucial in nutrition, as it is in many aspects of life

Balancing Oxalate Intake for Optimal Health

Balancing oxalate intake for optimal health is an important consideration for many individuals, particularly those prone to kidney stones or other health issues related to oxalate accumulation. Oxalates are naturally occurring compounds found in many plant-based foods, such as leafy greens, nuts, seeds, and some fruits and vegetables. While oxalates are not harmful for most people when consumed in moderation, they can contribute to health problems for some individuals, especially those with certain medical conditions.

1. **Understanding Oxalates**: Oxalates are compounds found in a variety of foods, particularly those that are plant-based. They are known to bind with minerals like calcium and form crystals, which can potentially lead to kidney stones in susceptible individuals. However, it's important to note that not everyone is sensitive to oxalates, and for many people, they are a natural and healthy part of their diet.

2. **Assessing Individual Sensitivity**: Some people may be more sensitive to oxalates than others. Factors such as genetics, gut health, and overall diet can influence how the body metabolizes and eliminates oxalates. Individuals who have a history of kidney stones, certain digestive disorders, or other health conditions may need to be more cautious about their oxalate intake.

3. **Balanced Diet Approach**: Rather than eliminating oxalate-rich foods from the diet, it's often more beneficial to focus on balance. Including a variety of foods in the diet ensures that you're getting a range of nutrients while also moderating oxalate intake. For example, if you enjoy spinach, which is high in oxalates, consider pairing it with foods lower in oxalates or higher in calcium to help offset its effects.

4. **Moderation is Key**: For most people, moderate consumption of oxalate-rich foods is unlikely to cause any issues. It's when these foods are consumed in excess or if someone is particularly sensitive to oxalates that problems may arise. Being mindful of portion sizes and not overdoing it on foods high in oxalates can help prevent potential health issues.

5. **Calcium Counterbalance**: Consuming foods high in calcium along with oxalate-rich foods

can help reduce the risk of oxalate crystals forming in the body. Calcium combines with oxalates in the digestive system, stopping their absorption into the bloodstream and potentially averting the formation of kidney stones. Foods like dairy products, fortified plant-based milk, and leafy greens (which are both high in calcium and contain oxalates) can be part of a balanced approach.

6. **Cooking and Preparation Methods:** Some cooking and preparation methods can help reduce the oxalate content of certain foods. For example, boiling or steaming vegetables can lower their oxalate content compared to eating them raw. Additionally, soaking nuts and seeds before consuming them can help reduce oxalate levels.

7. **Individualized Approach**: Individuals need to listen to their bodies and pay attention to how they respond to different foods. Keeping a food diary and noting any symptoms or reactions can help identify patterns and determine if certain foods high in oxalates are problematic for you.

8. **Consulting with a Healthcare Professional:** For individuals with specific health concerns related to oxalates, consulting with a healthcare professional, such as a registered dietitian or a nephrologist, can provide personalized guidance. They can help develop a dietary plan that balances oxalate intake with other nutritional needs and health considerations.

Balancing oxalate intake for optimal health involves understanding individual sensitivity, adopting a balanced diet approach, consuming oxalate-rich foods in moderation, considering calcium counterbalance, utilizing appropriate cooking and preparation methods, taking an individualized approach, and seeking guidance from healthcare professionals when needed. By being mindful of oxalate intake and making informed dietary choices, individuals can support their overall health and well-being

23

CHAPTER TWO

How To Eat A Diet Low In Oxalate

Diets low in oxalates include consuming fewer foods rich in oxalates. Certain kinds of fruits, vegetables, nuts, grains, and legumes are among the foods rich in oxalates. The majority of medical professionals suggest keeping oxalate consumption to less than 40–50 mg per day, while recommendations might vary.

Your diet should mostly consist of items like proteins, dairy products, white grains, and fruits and vegetables with low oxalate content if you want to keep within this limit. Certain vegetables and legumes may have their oxalate level decreased by soaking and boiling them.

Additionally, some medical professionals may advise changing your diet to include more foods high in calcium, less salt, and more water. Reducing your consumption of oxalates—found in certain fruits, vegetables, grains, legumes, and nuts—is the goal of low-oxalate diets.

What To Consume and Steer Clear Of

Foods are often classified into four groups according to the amount of oxalates they contain:

- **Extremely high**: above 100 mg per serving
- **High**: 26–99 mg per serving
- **Low**: 5–9 mg per serving
- **Moderate**: 10–25 mg per serving

When following a low-oxalate diet, you should avoid high-oxalate meals and beverages and eat mostly items with low to moderate levels of oxalate. foods to consume You may include a variety of naturally low-oxalate foods in a healthy, low-oxalate diet.

On a low-oxalate diet, you may consume the following foods.

Fruits:

- Apples
- Apricots
- Lemons
- Peaches
- Cherries
- Strawberries
- Bananas
- Blackberries
- Blueberries
- Apples

Grains and Starches:

- White rice
- Maize flour
- Oat bran

Vegetables:

- Mustard greens
- Broccoli
- Cabbage

- Cauliflower
- Mushrooms
- Onions
- Peas
- Zucchini

Proteins:

- Eggs
- Meat
- Fish,
- Poultry

Dairy products:

- Yogurt
- Cheese
- Milk
- Butter

Coffee, water, and fruit juice are some of the beverages.

Herbs and spices include cumin, dill, cilantro, and cinnamon.

Foods To Stay Away From

Foods rich in oxalates, such as certain fruits, vegetables, nuts, seeds, and grains, are restricted in a low-oxalate diet.

A low-oxalate diet prohibits the following foods:

- **Fruits**: raspberries, oranges, tangerines, kiwis, dates, and rhubarb

- **Legumes**: navy beans, fava beans, kidney beans, refried beans;

- **Nuts:** almonds, walnuts, macadamia nuts, cashews;

- **Vegetables**: spinach, chard, potatoes, beets, turnips, yams, okra, carrots

- **Seeds**: pumpkin and sunflower seeds

- Drinks: tomato juice, tea, hot chocolate, and chocolate milk;

- **Grains and starches**: corn grits, bulgur, brown rice, couscous, millet, and bulgur;

- Soy products, such as burgers, soybeans, and tofu

Keep in mind that soaking and boiling may drastically lower the amount of oxalate in a lot of veggies and legumes. Many fruits, vegetables, nuts, seeds, grains, and legumes that are rich in oxalates are restricted to a low-oxalate diet.

Does it aid in kidney stone prevention? According to some studies, consuming more oxalate may result in more oxalate being excreted in the urine, which may lead to the formation of kidney stones. On the other hand, boosting your calcium consumption could be a useful strategy for kidney stone prevention. This method offers an option to completely cut out foods rich in oxalate. Increasing your calcium intake may help your body absorb less oxalate, thus reducing the risk of kidney stones developing.

Even when participants were reaching the daily recommended intake for calcium, ingesting excessive levels of oxalate did not raise the chance of developing calcium oxalate kidney stones, according to 10-person research. But given the tiny sample size of this study, additional research on this subject is required by experts.

The recommended daily allowance of calcium is **1,000–1,200 mg,** which is found in foods such as dairy products, leafy greens, sardines, and seeds. Other methods to lower the risk of kidney stones caused by calcium oxalate include the following:

- **Consume less salt**: Research indicates that eating a lot of salt may increase your chance of getting kidney stones.
- **Steer clear of vitamin C pills**: If your doctor does not advise you to use high-dose vitamin C pills, stay away from them since your body will turn them into oxalate.

- **Continue to drink water**: You may lower your risk of kidney stones and enhance urine production by increasing your fluid intake.

  Getting enough calcium in your diet may have the same impact as limiting oxalate in your diet when it comes to reducing oxalate excretion in urine. Many assert that oxalates might be linked to various health issues, such as autism. Indeed, tiny research discovered that when compared to a control group, children with autism had far higher blood and urine oxalate levels. Nevertheless, there is no evidence to support the theory that dietary oxalates cause autism or to support the idea that treating autism with a low-oxalate diet may be beneficial.

  Low oxalate diets have also been used to treat vulvodynia, a disorder that causes persistent vulva discomfort. Research indicates that there is no correlation between consuming dietary oxalate and an increased incidence of vulvodynia. A low-oxalate diet, however, could support pain management. There is no proof that oxalate ingestion directly causes autism or vulvodynia, despite some people's claims to the contrary.

33

CHAPTER THREE

Foods High In Oxalate

When reducing oxalate consumption, these foods have to be stayed away from. Foods classified as high oxalate often have a serving size of 10 mg or higher. Plants contain oxalates.

Foods with the highest oxalate content include:

- Fruits
- Vegetables
- Nuts
- Seeds
- Some legumes
- Grains

High-oxalate fruits include:

- Berries
- Kiwis
- Figs
- Purple grapes

Some vegetables that are high in oxalate include:

- Potatoes
- Rhubarb
- Leeks
- Spinach
- Beets
- Swiss chard

Avoid the following to lower your intake of oxalate:

- Almonds
- Cashews
- Peanuts
- Soy products

Moreover, oxalate content is high in some grain products, such as:

- Bran flakes
- Wheat germ
- Quinoa

Foods that are high in oxalates include the following:

- Cocoa
- Chocolate
- Tea

Although it can seem like oxalate is present in a lot of meals, not everything has to be avoided. You may eat foods containing oxalate as long as you prepare ahead and maintain a balanced diet with appropriate quantity limits. It is essential to discuss what you can and cannot eat to suit your requirements with your doctor or a nutritionist. Dairy doesn't include oxalate; nonetheless, be mindful of salt levels (think cheese) and oxalate-containing foods like chocolate and cacao.

Foods High In Calcium

Urine oxalate levels may be lowered by increasing calcium intake while consuming oxalate-containing meals. Select dairy products like milk, yogurt, and cheese that are rich in calcium. Additionally, vegetables may be a rich source of calcium. To raise your calcium levels, choose one of the following foods:

- Broccoli
- Watercress
- Kale
- Okra

Legumes with a high calcium content and a moderate calcium content are:

- Kidney beans
- Chickpeas
- Baked beans
- Navy beans

Among the fish high in calcium are:

- Sardines with bones
- Whitebait
- Salmon

Because meats don't contain oxalate, they are safe to consume. However, consuming a lot of food might make kidney stones more likely. Remember to eat no more than two to three servings, or four to six ounces, every day.

How To Prevent Kidney Stones

Add a high-calcium item to a meal that also includes food that has higher oxalate levels to reduce your chance of kidney stones. It's more crucial to concentrate on matching a high-calcium dish with a high-oxalate food before examining the nutrients separately.

It may be necessary to add a second source of calcium since many meals have a high oxalate content in addition to a modest amount of calcium. For instance, be sure to include some milk in your oatmeal if you include wheat germ. Don't feel bad if you prepare spinach and serve it with lasagna or pizza. To assist in maintaining balance, mix in some Greek or normal yogurt if you're seeking a berry smoothie.

From Whence Does Oxalate Originate?

Many of the items in our diets contain oxalate. The primary food sources of oxalate include:

- Spinach and other green, leafy vegetables
- Rhubarb
- Wheat bran
- Almonds
- Beets
- Navy beans
- Chocolate
- Okra
- French fries and baked potatoes
- Nuts and seeds
- Soy products
- Tea
- Strawberries and raspberries

Your GI tract breaks down these meals and absorbs the nutrients when you consume them. The residual wastes next make their way to your kidneys, where they are eliminated into your urine. Oxalic acid is the byproduct of oxalate degradation. In the urine, it may react with calcium to generate calcium oxalate crystals.

What Signs and Symptoms Are Present?

Until kidney stones begin to pass through your urinary system, they may not produce any symptoms. The discomfort may be excruciating when stones shift. The following are the main signs of calcium oxalate crystals in the urine: intense, sometimes wave-like pain in your side and back; pain when you urinate; blood in your urine, which can appear red, pink, or brown; cloudy urine; foul-smelling urine; nausea and vomiting; fever and chills if you have an infection

Why Do Crystals of Calcium Oxalate Form?

Chemicals in urine often prevent oxalate from crystallizing and adhering to one another. Urine, however, may crystallize and create stones if you have too little or too much oxalate in it. Some causes of this include:

- *Consuming a diet heavy in protein, salt, or oxalate*

- *Not drinking enough water (being dehydrated)*

In some instances, the crystals turn into stones as a result of an underlying illness. The following conditions increase your risk of developing calcium oxalate stones:

- Hyperparathyroidism, or an excess of parathyroid hormone;

- Inflammatory bowel disease (IBD), including ulcerative colitis and Crohn's disease.

- Dental disease, an inherited kidney-damaging condition; and gastric bypass surgery for weight loss.
- obesity
- Diabetes

43

CHAPTER FOUR

How Are They Identified?

To determine if you have calcium oxalate stones, your doctor may do the following tests:

Urine test: To measure the amount of oxalate in your urine, your doctor could ask for a 24-hour urine sample. For a whole day, you will need to collect pee throughout the day. Less than 45 mg of oxalate per day is considered normal in the urine.

A blood test: Your blood may be tested by your doctor to check for the Dent disease-causing gene mutation.

Imaging examinations: Kidney stones may be seen on an X-ray or CT scan.

What Takes Place When a Woman Is Pregnant?

Blood flow rises throughout pregnancy to support your developing kid. Your kidneys filter more blood, which results in more oxalate being eliminated from your urine. Extra oxalate in your urine might encourage the creation of kidney stones, even though your risk of developing kidney stones is the same during pregnancy as it is at other periods of your life.

Pregnancy problems may arise from kidney stones. According to some research, stones increase preeclampsia and cesarean birth. Imaging examinations such as CT scans and X-rays may not be healthy for your unborn child during pregnancy. Instead, your doctor may diagnose you using an ultrasound.

During pregnancy, up to 84% of stones move through on their own. After birth, around half of the stones that do not pass during pregnancy will do so. Procedures like a stent or lithotripsy may remove the kidney stone if you are experiencing significant symptoms from it or if you might lose your pregnancy.

How Is the Condition Being Treated?

Without medical intervention, small stones may naturally disappear in four to six weeks. If you drink more water, it will aid in flushing out the stone. Additionally, your physician may recommend an alpha-blocker such as tamsulosin (Flomax) or doxazosin (Cardura). These medications assist the stone exiting your kidney more rapidly by relaxing your ureter. Until the stone passes, painkillers like acetaminophen (Tylenol) and ibuprofen (Advil, Motrin) might help you feel better. However, before using non-steroidal anti-inflammatory medications (ibuprofen, naproxen, aspirin, and celecoxib) if you are pregnant, see your doctor.

To remove the stone, you may need to use one of the following methods if it's particularly big or doesn't go away on its own:

- Shock wave lithotripsy administered externally (ESWL). The stone is broken into little bits by ESWL using sound waves that are delivered from outside your body. You should be able to pass the stone bits in your urine a few weeks following ESWL.

- Ultrateroscopy. During this surgery, your doctor will insert a narrow scope into your bladder and insert the end containing a camera into your kidney. Subsequently, the stone is either taken out using a basket or broken up using a laser or other equipment before being taken out. To hold the ureter open and enable urine to drain while you recuperate, the surgeon could insert a stent, which is a tiny plastic tube.

- Nephrolithotomy by percutaneous means. Under general anesthesia, this surgery is performed while you are pain-free and unconscious. Your surgeon will create a little incision in your back and use tiny equipment to remove the stone.

How can crystals of calcium oxalate be avoided?

By using these suggestions, you may prevent kidney stones and calcium oxalate from crystallizing in your urine:

- Sip more water. For those who have had kidney stones, several medical professionals advise consuming 2.6 quarts (2.5 liters) of water daily. Find out from your doctor how much fluid is appropriate for you.

- Reduce the amount of salt you eat. A diet heavy in salt may raise the calcium content of your urine, which can promote the formation of stones.

- Restrict your consumption of protein. A balanced diet must include enough protein, but not too much. Stones may develop if this vitamin is consumed in excess. Protein should make up no more than 30% of your daily caloric intake.

- Make sure your diet has the appropriate quantity of calcium. Increased amounts of oxalate might result from a diet low in calcium. Make sure you're receiving the right quantity of calcium each day for your age to avoid this. The best sources of calcium are dairy products and cheese. Kidney stones have been related by some to calcium supplements when they are not taken with a meal.

- Reduce your intake of foods rich in oxalate, such as nuts, rhubarb, bran, soy, and beets. When you do consume meals high in oxalate, pair them with a calcium-containing beverage, such as milk. This will prevent the oxalate from crystallizing in your urine by binding to calcium before it reaches your kidneys. Find out more about a diet low in oxalate.

Many wholesome and nutrient-dense foods, such as certain kinds of fruits, vegetables, nuts, seeds, and carbohydrates, are off-limits in low-oxalate diets. For instance, spinach has a high oxalate content but is also a fantastic source of calcium, magnesium, fiber, and vitamin A. In the same way, beets are rich in essential elements like manganese, potassium, and folate but also high in oxalates.

Because a low oxalate diet excludes so many items, it may also be difficult for those with certain dietary requirements or preferences. Particularly vegans and vegetarians may struggle to get enough protein due to the high oxalates found in plant-based protein sources such as beans, almonds, and tofu. Many detrimental side effects, such as reduced immunity, weakness, anemia, and stunted development, may result from a protein deficit. As a result, if you adopt a low-oxalate diet, you must make sure the diet provides for all of your nutritional requirements.

Plenty of healthful foods include a lot of oxalates. For vegans and vegetarians, maintaining a low-oxalate diet might be difficult since oxalates are present in a lot of plant-based protein sources.

CHAPTER FIVE

Low -Oxalates Plans and Recipes

Here are some meal plans and recipes that are relatively low in oxalates:

Breakfast:

Spinach and Feta Omelette

Ingredients:

- 2 eggs
- Handful of fresh spinach
- 1 tablespoon crumbled feta cheese
- Salt and pepper to taste

Preparation:

1. Combine the eggs in a bowl and whisk until they are thoroughly mixed, then season with salt and pepper according to your taste preferences.

2. Sauté spinach in a pan until wilted, then add the whisked eggs.

3. Once the eggs are mostly set, sprinkle feta cheese over one half and fold the other half over the top.

4. Continue cooking until the cheese has melted completely and the eggs are thoroughly cooked.

Low-Oxalate Smoothie

Ingredients:

- 1 cup unsweetened almond milk

- 1/2 cup frozen blueberries

- 1/2 ripe banana

- 1 tablespoon almond butter

- 1 scoop protein powder (optional)

Preparation:

Blend all ingredients until smooth.

Lunch:

Grilled Chicken and Vegetable Salad

Ingredients:

- Grilled chicken breast
- Mixed salad greens (lettuce, arugula, etc.)
- Sliced cucumber
- Cherry tomatoes
- Sliced bell peppers
- Balsamic vinaigrette dressing (low-oxalate)

Preparation:

1. Grill chicken breast until fully cooked.
2. Assemble salad with mixed greens, cucumber, tomatoes, and bell peppers.
3. Cut the grilled chicken into slices and arrange them atop the salad.

Drizzle With Balsamic Vinaigrette Dressing

Lentil Soup

Ingredients:

- 1 cup dried lentils (rinsed)
- 1 onion (chopped)
- 2 carrots (chopped)

- 2 celery stalks (chopped)
- 2 cloves garlic (minced)
- 4 cups vegetable broth
- 1 teaspoon cumin
- 1 teaspoon paprika
- Salt and pepper to taste

Preparation:

1. In a large pot, sauté onion, carrots, celery, and garlic until softened.
2. Add lentils, vegetable broth, cumin, paprika, salt, and pepper.
3. Bring to a boil, then reduce heat and simmer for about 30-40 minutes, or until lentils are tender.

Dinner:

Baked Salmon with Steamed Broccoli

Ingredients:

- Salmon fillets
- Lemon slices

- Salt and pepper to taste

- Olive oil

- Broccoli florets

Preparation:

1. Preheat oven to 375°F (190°C).

2. Arrange the salmon fillets on a baking sheet that's been lined with parchment paper.

3. Season salmon with salt, and pepper, and drizzle with olive oil. Place lemon slices on top.

4. Bake until the salmon is thoroughly cooked, typically for 12 to 15 minutes.

5. While the salmon is baking, steam broccoli until tender-crisp.

6. Serve salmon with steamed broccoli on the side.

Turkey and Vegetable Stir-Fry

Ingredients:

- Turkey breast slices

- Assorted vegetables (bell peppers, snap peas, broccoli, carrots, etc.)

- Soy sauce (low-sodium)

- Garlic powder

- Ginger powder

- Sesame oil

Preparation:

1. Heat sesame oil in a large skillet or wok over medium-high heat.

2. Proceed to add turkey breast slices and cook them until they achieve a golden brown color.

3. Add assorted vegetables and stir-fry until tender-crisp.

4. Season with garlic powder, ginger powder, and soy sauce to taste.

5. Scrve hot.

Breakfast:

Quinoa Breakfast Bowl

Ingredients:

- Cooked quinoa

- Sliced avocado

- Diced tomatoes

- Crumbled goat cheese

- Poached egg (optional)

Preparation:

1. Cook quinoa according to package instructions.

2. In a bowl, layer cooked quinoa with sliced avocado, diced tomatoes, and crumbled goat cheese.

3. Top with a poached egg if desired.

Greek Yogurt Parfait

Ingredients:

- Greek yogurt (unsweetened)
- Fresh berries (blueberries, strawberries, raspberries)
- Chia seeds
- Almonds (chopped)
- Honey (optional)

Preparation:

1. In a glass or bowl, layer Greek yogurt with fresh berries, chia seeds, and chopped almonds.
2. Drizzle with honey if desired.

Lunch:

Turkey and Avocado Wrap

Ingredients:

- Sliced turkey breast
- Whole wheat tortilla
- Sliced avocado

- Mixed greens

- Mustard or hummus (optional)

Preparation:

1. Lay the whole wheat tortilla flat.

2. Layer sliced turkey breast, avocado, mixed greens, and a spread of mustard or hummus if desired.

3. Roll up the tortilla tightly and slice it in half.

Cauliflower Rice Sushi Rolls

Ingredients:

- Nori seaweed sheets

- Cauliflower rice

- Sliced cucumber

- Sliced avocado

- Cooked shrimp or imitation crab (optional)

Preparation:

1. Lay a nori seaweed sheet flat on a bamboo sushi mat or clean surface.

2. Spread a thin layer of cauliflower rice over the nori sheet, leaving a border around the edges.

3. Arrange sliced cucumber, avocado, and cooked shrimp or imitation crab in a line along the bottom edge of the nori sheet.

4. Roll the nori sheet tightly, using the bamboo sushi mat to help guide the rolling process.

5. Slice the sushi roll into bite-sized pieces and serve with soy sauce or tamari for dipping.

Dinner:

Grilled Lemon Herb Chicken with Asparagus

Ingredients:

1. Chicken breasts

2. Lemon juice

3. Freshly chopped herbs like parsley, thyme, and rosemary

4. Salt and pepper to taste

5. Asparagus spears

Preparation:

1. In a bowl, mix lemon juice, chopped fresh herbs, salt, and pepper.

2. Marinate chicken breasts in the lemon herb mixture for at least 30 minutes.

3. Preheat the grill to medium-high heat.

4. Cook the chicken breasts on the grill for 6 to 8 minutes on each side, or until they are fully cooked.

5. While the chicken is grilling, toss asparagus spears with olive oil, salt, and pepper.

6. Grill asparagus spears for 4-5 minutes, or until tender-crisp.

7. Serve grilled chicken with grilled asparagus on the side.

Zucchini Noodles with Pesto Sauce

Ingredients:

- Zucchini

- Cherry tomatoes (halved)

- Pesto sauce (homemade or store-bought, low-oxalate)
- Grated Parmesan cheese (optional)

Preparation:

1. Use a spiralizer to spiralize zucchini into noodles.

2. Heat a skillet over medium heat and add zucchini noodles and cherry tomatoes.

3. Sauté for 2-3 minutes, or until zucchini noodles are just tender.

4. Take off the heat and mix thoroughly with pesto sauce.

5. You may choose to add grated Parmesan cheese as a finishing touch before serving.

Breakfast:

Buckwheat Pancakes

Ingredients:

- 1 cup buckwheat flour
- 1 tablespoon sugar

- 1 teaspoon baking powder
- Pinch of salt
- 1 cup almond milk
- 1 egg
- 1 tablespoon melted coconut oil

Preparation:

1. In a mixing bowl, whisk together buckwheat flour, sugar, baking powder, and salt.

2. In another bowl, whisk almond milk, egg, and melted coconut oil.

3. Combine the wet ingredients with the dry ones and stir until they're thoroughly mixed. Next, warm up a skillet over medium heat and lightly coat it with coconut oil.

4. Pour batter onto the skillet to form pancakes and cook until bubbles form on the surface, then flip and cook until golden brown on both sides.

5. Serve with fresh fruit and maple syrup.

Tofu Scramble

Ingredients:

- Firm tofu
- Diced bell peppers
- Diced onions
- Spinach
- Turmeric powder
- Garlic powder
- Salt and pepper to taste

Preparation:

1. Press tofu to remove excess moisture, then crumble it into a bowl.

2. Sauté diced bell peppers and onions in a skillet until softened.

3. Add crumbled tofu to the skillet and season with turmeric powder, garlic powder, salt, and pepper.

4. Cook until tofu is heated through and slightly golden, then stir in spinach until wilted.

5. Serve hot with whole grain toast or on its own.

Lunch:

Caprese Salad

Ingredients:

- Sliced tomatoes
- Sliced fresh mozzarella cheese
- Fresh basil leaves
- Balsamic glaze (low-oxalate)
- Olive oil
- Salt and pepper to taste

Preparation:

1. Place slices of tomatoes and fresh mozzarella cheese alternately on a plate.
2. Place fresh basil leaves amidst the tomato and cheese slices
3. Drizzle with balsamic glaze and olive oil, then season with salt and pepper.

4. Serve as a refreshing salad.

Lentil and Vegetable Stir-Fry

Ingredients:

- Cooked lentils
- Assorted vegetables (broccoli, bell peppers, snap peas, carrots, etc.)
- Soy sauce (low-sodium)
- Sesame oil
- Garlic powder
- Ginger powder

Preparation:

1. Warm sesame oil in a spacious skillet or wok on medium-high heat.
2. Add assorted vegetables and stir-fry until tender-crisp.
3. Mix the cooked lentils into the skillet, ensuring they're evenly distributed.

4. Season with soy sauce, garlic powder, and ginger powder to taste.

5. Continue cooking for an additional minute or until thoroughly heated.

6. Serve hot with brown rice or quinoa.

Dinner:

Baked Cod with Lemon Herb Butter

Ingredients:

- Cod fillets

- Lemon juice

- Freshly chopped herbs like parsley, dill, and chives

- Butter or ghee

- Salt and pepper to taste

Preparation:

1. Preheat oven to 375°F (190°C).

2. Arrange cod fillets on a baking sheet that has been lined with parchment paper.

3. Drizzle lemon juice over the cod fillets, then season with chopped fresh herbs, salt, and pepper.
4. Place a small piece of butter or ghee on top of each cod fillet.
5. Bake for 15-20 minutes, or until fish is cooked through and flakes easily with a fork.
6. Enjoy it piping hot alongside steamed vegetables or a fresh side salad.

Spaghetti Squash with Marinara Sauce

Ingredients:

- Spaghetti squash
- Marinara sauce (low-oxalate)
- Fresh basil leaves
- Grated Parmesan cheese (optional)

Preparation:

1. Preheat oven to 400°F (200°C).

2. Slice the spaghetti squash lengthwise and remove the seeds from the center.

3. Place spaghetti squash halves cut side down on a baking sheet lined with parchment paper.

4. Bake for 40-45 minutes, or until squash is tender and easily pierced with a fork.

5. Use a fork to scrape the cooked spaghetti squash into strands.

6. Heat marinara sauce in a saucepan over medium heat, then stir in spaghetti squash until heated through.

7. Serve hot with fresh basil leaves and grated Parmesan cheese on top if desired.

Breakfast:

Sweet Potato Hash

Ingredients:

- Sweet potatoes (peeled and diced)
- Diced bell peppers

- Diced onions

- Cooked chicken sausage (sliced)

- Olive oil

- Paprika

- Salt and pepper to taste

Preparation:

1. Warm up some olive oil in a skillet on medium heat.

2. Add diced sweet potatoes and cook until slightly browned and softened.

3. Add diced bell peppers, onions, and sliced chicken sausage to the skillet.

4. Season with paprika, salt, and pepper.

5. Continue cooking until the vegetables are soft and the sausage is thoroughly heated.

6. Serve hot, optionally topped with a fried egg.

Cottage Cheese and Fruit Bowl

Ingredients:

- Cottage cheese

- Fresh fruit (such as pineapple, kiwi, and mango)

- Chopped nuts (such as almonds or walnuts)

- Honey (optional)

Preparation:

1. Spoon cottage cheese into a bowl.

2. Top with diced fresh fruit and chopped nuts.

3. Drizzle with honey if desired.

Lunch:

Turkey and Spinach Salad

- Ingredients:

- Sliced turkey breast

- Baby spinach leaves

- Sliced strawberries

- Sliced almonds

- Balsamic vinaigrette dressing (low-oxalate)

Preparation:

1. Arrange baby spinach leaves on a plate.
2. Top with sliced turkey breast, sliced strawberries, and sliced almonds.
3. Drizzle with balsamic vinaigrette dressing.
4. Eggplant and Tomato Stacks

Ingredients:

- Eggplant (sliced into rounds)
- Sliced tomatoes
- Fresh mozzarella cheese slices
- Fresh basil leaves
- Balsamic glaze (low-oxalate)

Preparation:

1. Preheat oven to 400°F (200°C).
2. Arrange slices of eggplant on a baking sheet that has been lined with parchment paper.

3. Top each eggplant round with a slice of tomato, a slice of fresh mozzarella cheese, and a basil leaf.

4. Drizzle with balsamic glaze.

5. Bake until the cheese is melted and bubbly, typically around 15 to 20 minutes.

6. Serve hot as a flavorful appetizer or light lunch.

Dinner:

Shrimp Stir-Fry with Snow Peas

Ingredients:

- Shrimp (peeled and deveined)
- Snow peas
- Sliced bell peppers
- Sliced carrots
- Soy sauce (low-sodium)
- Garlic powder
- Ginger powder
- Sesame oil

Preparation:

1. Warm sesame oil in a spacious skillet or wok on medium-high heat.
2. Place the shrimp in the skillet and cook until they turn pink and become opaque.
3. Add snow peas, sliced bell peppers, and sliced carrots to the skillet.
4. Stir-fry until vegetables are tender-crisp.
5. Season with soy sauce, garlic powder, and ginger powder to taste.
6. Continue cooking for an additional minute or until thoroughly heated.
7. Serve hot with steamed rice or noodles.

Stuffed Bell Peppers with Ground Turkey

Ingredients:

- Bell peppers (halved and seeds removed)
- Ground turkey
- Cooked quinoa

- Diced tomatoes

- Chopped onions

- Minced garlic

- Italian seasoning

- Salt and pepper to taste

Preparation:

1. Preheat oven to 375°F (190°C).

2. In a skillet, cook ground turkey until browned, then drain any excess fat.

3. Add diced tomatoes, chopped onions, minced garlic, Italian seasoning, salt, and pepper to the skillet, and cook until vegetables are softened.

4. Stir in cooked quinoa until well combined.

5. Stuff bell pepper halves with the turkey and quinoa mixture.

6. Place stuffed bell peppers in a baking dish and cover with foil.

7. Bake until the peppers are tender, typically for 25 to 30 minutes.

8. Serve hot as a satisfying dinner option.

Breakfast:

Banana Oatmeal Pancakes

Ingredients:

- 1 ripe banana

- 1/2 cup rolled oats

- 1/4 cup almond milk

- 1 egg

- 1/2 teaspoon vanilla extract

- Pinch of cinnamon

Preparation:

1. In a blender, combine banana, rolled oats, almond milk, egg, vanilla extract, and cinnamon.

2. Blend until smooth.

3. Preheat a non-stick skillet over medium heat and lightly coat it with oil or cooking spray.

4. Pour the pancake batter onto the skillet to create pancakes.

5. Cook until bubbles start to form on the surface, then flip and continue cooking until both sides are golden brown.

6. Serve warm with your favorite toppings such as fresh fruit or maple syrup.

Veggie Egg Muffins

Ingredients:

- Eggs
- Diced bell peppers
- Diced onions
- Diced tomatoes
- Spinach leaves
- Salt and pepper to taste

Preparation:

1. Preheat oven to 350°F (175°C) and grease a muffin tin.

2. In a bowl, whisk together eggs, diced bell peppers, onions, tomatoes, spinach leaves, salt, and pepper.

3. Pour the egg mixture into the muffin tin, ensuring each cup is filled to about 3/4 capacity.

4. Bake for 20-25 minutes, or until the egg muffins are firm and display a golden brown color.

5. Allow to cool slightly before serving.

Lunch:

Tuna Salad Lettuce Wraps

Ingredients:

- Canned tuna (drained)
- Diced celery
- Diced red onion
- Diced pickles
- Dijon mustard
- Greek yogurt (unsweetened)
- Lettuce leaves

Preparation:

1. In a bowl, combine canned tuna, diced celery, diced red onion, diced pickles, Dijon mustard, and Greek yogurt.

2. Mix until well combined.

3. Spoon the tuna salad onto lettuce leaves and wrap to form lettuce wraps.

4. Provide a lunch choice that is light and refreshing.

Quinoa Salad with Lemon Vinaigrette

Ingredients:

- Cooked quinoa
- Diced cucumber
- Cherry tomatoes (halved)
- Diced bell peppers
- Chopped fresh parsley
- Lemon juice
- Olive oil

- Salt and pepper to taste

Preparation:

1. In a large bowl, combine cooked quinoa, diced cucumber, cherry tomatoes, diced bell peppers, and chopped fresh parsley.

2. Combine lemon juice, olive oil, salt, and pepper in a small bowl to create the vinaigrette.

3. Drizzle the vinaigrette over the quinoa salad and mix until evenly coated.

4. Serve chilled as a nutritious and satisfying lunch.

Dinner:

Baked Chicken with Roasted Vegetables

Ingredients:

- Chicken thighs or breasts
- Assorted vegetables (such as carrots, potatoes, and Brussels sprouts)
- Olive oil
- Garlic powder

- Paprika
- Salt and pepper to taste

Preparation:

1. Preheat oven to 400°F (200°C).
2. Place chicken and assorted vegetables on a baking sheet lined with parchment paper.
3. Drizzle olive oil over the chicken and vegetables, then sprinkle with garlic powder, paprika, salt, and pepper.
4. Toss to coat evenly.
5. Bake until the chicken is thoroughly cooked and the vegetables are tender, which typically takes 25 to 30 minutes.
6. Serve hot as a hearty and flavorful dinner.

Turkey and Quinoa Stuffed Bell Peppers

Ingredients:

- Bell peppers (halved and seeds removed)
- Ground turkey

- Cooked quinoa

- Diced tomatoes

- Chopped onions

- Minced garlic

- Italian seasoning

- Salt and pepper to taste

Preparation:

1. Preheat oven to 375°F (190°C).

2. In a skillet, cook ground turkey until browned, then drain any excess fat.

3. Add diced tomatoes, chopped onions, minced garlic, Italian seasoning, salt, and pepper to the skillet, and cook until vegetables are softened.

4. Stir in cooked quinoa until well combined.

5. Stuff bell pepper halves with the turkey and quinoa mixture.

6. Place stuffed bell peppers in a baking dish and cover with foil.

7. Bake until the peppers are tender, typically taking 25-30 minutes. Serve while hot as a nourishing and fulfilling dinner choice.

Breakfast:

Nut butter and berry Greek yogurt bowl

Ingredients:

- Greek yogurt (unsweetened)
- Nut butter (almond, cashew, or peanut)
- Fresh berries (strawberries, blueberries, raspberries)
- Honey (optional)

Preparation:

- Spoon Greek yogurt into a bowl.
- Swirl in a dollop of nut butter.
- Arrange fresh berries on top and optionally drizzle with honey.

- Mix well and enjoy a creamy and satisfying breakfast bowl.
- Spinach and Mushroom Frittata

Ingredients:

- Eggs
- Fresh spinach leaves
- Sliced mushrooms
- Diced onions
- Olive oil
- Salt and pepper to taste

Preparation:

1. Preheat oven to 350°F (175°C).
2. In a skillet, sauté sliced mushrooms and diced onions in olive oil until softened.
3. Toss fresh spinach leaves into the skillet and cook until they wilt. Combine eggs, salt, and pepper in a separate bowl, whisking until well blended.

4. . Pour the egg mixture over the vegetables in the skillet and cook on the stovetop until the edges start to firm up, which should only take a few minutes.

5. Transfer the skillet to the oven and bake for 10-15 minutes, or until the frittata is set in the center.

6. Slice and serve warm.

Lunch:

Tofu and Vegetable Stir-Fry

Ingredients:

- Firm tofu (cubed)

- Assorted vegetables (such as broccoli, bell peppers, carrots, and snap peas)

- Soy sauce (low-sodium)

- Garlic powder

- Ginger powder

- Sesame oil

Preparation:

1. Heat sesame oil in a sizable skillet or wok over medium-high heat.

2. Introduce cubed tofu into the skillet, cooking until it achieves a light golden brown.

3. Incorporate an assortment of vegetables into the skillet, stir-frying until they reach a tender-crisp texture.

4. Season to taste with soy sauce, garlic powder, and ginger powder.

5. Continue cooking for an additional minute or until thoroughly heated.

6. Serve hot with brown rice or quinoa.

Lentil and Kale Salad

Ingredients:

- Cooked lentils
- Chopped kale leaves
- Diced cucumber

- Cherry tomatoes (halved)

- Crumbled feta cheese

- Lemon juice

- Olive oil

- Salt and pepper to taste

Preparation:

1. In a large bowl, combine cooked lentils, chopped kale leaves, diced cucumber, cherry tomatoes, and crumbled feta cheese.

2. In a small bowl, whisk together lemon juice, olive oil, salt, and pepper to make the dressing.

3. Drizzle the dressing onto the salad and mix thoroughly until everything is evenly coated.

4. Serve chilled as a nutritious and flavorful lunch option.

Dinner:

Baked Salmon with Herb Crust

Ingredients:

- Salmon fillets

- Herbs that have just been chopped, such as parsley, dill, and chives.

- Lemon zest

- Olive oil

- Salt and pepper to taste

Preparation:

1. Preheat oven to 400°F (200°C).

2. Arrange the salmon fillets on a baking sheet that's been covered with parchment paper.

3. In a small bowl, mix chopped fresh herbs, lemon zest, olive oil, salt, and pepper to form a paste.

4. Spread the herb mixture evenly over the salmon fillets.

5. Bake until the salmon is fully cooked and easily flakes with a fork, typically taking 12 to 15 minutes.

6. Serve hot with your favorite side dishes.

Stir-fried shrimp with Broccoli and Cashews

Ingredients:

- Shrimp (peeled and deveined)
- Broccoli florets
- Cashews (unsalted)
- Soy sauce (low-sodium)
- Garlic powder
- Ginger powder
- Sesame oil

Preparation:

1. Heat sesame oil in a spacious skillet or wok over medium-high heat.

2. Introduce shrimp to the skillet and cook until they turn pink and opaque.

3. Add broccoli florets and cashews to the skillet, and stir-fry until the broccoli reaches a tender-crisp texture.

4. Season with soy sauce, garlic powder, and ginger powder according to your taste preferences.

5. Allow it to cook for an additional minute or until everything is heated through.

6. Serve hot with steamed rice or noodles.

Breakfast:

Chia Seed Pudding

Ingredients:

1. 1/4 cup chia seeds

2. Use 1 cup of your preferred milk, such as unsweetened almond milk.

3. Add 1 tablespoon of maple syrup or your desired sweetener

4. Fresh fruit for topping (such as sliced strawberries, blueberries, or kiwi)

Preparation:

1. In a bowl or jar, mix chia seeds, almond milk, and maple syrup.
2. Allow it to rest in the refrigerator for a minimum of 2 hours, or overnight until it reaches a pudding-like thickness.

Veggie Breakfast Burrito

Ingredients:

- Whole grain tortilla
- Scrambled eggs
- Sautéed bell peppers, onions, and spinach
- Salsa (low-oxalate)
- Avocado slices

Preparation:

1. Warm up the tortilla in a skillet or microwave.

2. Layer scrambled eggs, sautéed vegetables, salsa, and avocado slices onto the tortilla.

3. Roll it up into a burrito and serve warm.

Lunch:

Turkey and Avocado Salad

Ingredients:

- Sliced turkey breast

- Mixed salad greens (lettuce, spinach, arugula, etc.)

- Sliced avocado

- Cherry tomatoes

- Sliced cucumber

- Balsamic vinaigrette dressing (low-oxalate)

Preparation:

1. Arrange mixed salad greens on a plate.

2. Top with sliced turkey breast, avocado slices, cherry tomatoes, and sliced cucumber.

3. Drizzle with balsamic vinaigrette dressing.

Quinoa and Black Bean Bowl

Ingredients:

- Cooked quinoa

- Canned black beans (rinsed and drained)

- Diced bell peppers

- Diced red onions

- Chopped cilantro

- Lime juice

- Salt and pepper to taste

Preparation:

1. In a bowl, mix cooked quinoa, black beans, diced bell peppers, diced red onions, and chopped cilantro.

2. Drizzle with lime juice and season with salt and pepper.

3. Toss until well combined and serve at room temperature or chilled.

Dinner:

Grilled Chicken Skewers with Vegetable Medley

Ingredients:

- Chicken breast (cut into cubes)
- Cherry tomatoes
- Button mushrooms
- Zucchini (sliced)
- Red onion (cut into chunks)
- Olive oil

- Lemon juice
- Garlic powder
- Italian seasoning
- Salt and pepper to taste

Preparation:

1. Preheat the grill to medium-high heat.

2. Thread chicken cubes, cherry tomatoes, mushrooms, zucchini slices, and red onion chunks onto skewers.

3. In a small bowl, whisk together olive oil, lemon juice, garlic powder, Italian seasoning, salt, and pepper to make the marinade.

4. Brush the marinade over the skewers.

5. Grill skewers for 10-12 minutes, turning occasionally, until chicken is cooked through and vegetables are tender.

6. Serve hot with a side of rice or quinoa.

Cauliflower Rice Stir-Fry

Ingredients:

- Cauliflower rice
- Diced carrots
- Peas
- Diced bell peppers
- Diced onions
- Minced garlic
- Soy sauce (low-sodium)
- Sesame oil

Preparation:

1. Warm sesame oil in a spacious skillet or wok on medium heat.
2. Add diced carrots, peas, bell peppers, onions, and minced garlic to the skillet.
3. Stir-fry until vegetables are tender-crisp.

4. Partition the skillet by pushing the vegetables to one side, then introduce cauliflower rice to the opposite side.

5. Combine vegetables and cauliflower rice in the skillet and stir in soy sauce.

6. Cook for another minute, then serve hot.

Conclusion

A class of substances called oxalates may be found in many different foods, such as certain fruits, vegetables, grains, beans, and nuts. Kidney stones made of calcium oxalate may develop as a result of excessive oxalate excretion in the urine. Some try removing oxalate from their diets in an attempt to avoid this, since it may help reduce the chance of kidney stones. Reducing your oxalate intake may help reduce the chance of kidney stones if you have a high risk of developing them. The foods highest in

Navigating a low-oxalate diet doesn't have to be overwhelming. By understanding the role of oxalates in the body and adopting a balanced approach to your diet, you can optimize your health and reduce the risk of complications like kidney stones. Remember, moderation is key. Rather than completely avoiding oxalate-rich foods, focus on incorporating a variety of nutrient-rich options into your meals.

Pairing oxalate-rich foods with calcium-rich sources can also help mitigate their effects. If you have specific health concerns or conditions, consulting with a healthcare provider or dietitian can provide personalized guidance to ensure you're making the best choices for your well-being. With a little knowledge and mindful eating, you can support your health and enjoy a varied and delicious diet.